Hemochromatosis Diet for Beginners

A 4-Week Low-Iron Meal Plan with Easy Recipes to Reduce Iron Absorption, Alleviate Symptoms & Boost Energy Naturally

copyright © 2025 Larry Jamesonn

All rights reserved No part of this book may be reproduced, or stored in a retrieval system, or transmitted in any form or by any means, electronic, mechanical, photocopying, recording, or otherwise, without express written permission of the publisher.

Disclaimer

By reading this disclaimer, you are accepting the terms of the disclaimer in full. If you disagree with this disclaimer, please do not read the guide.

All of the content within this guide is provided for informational and educational purposes only, and should not be accepted as independent medical or other professional advice. The author is not a doctor, physician, nurse, mental health provider, or registered nutritionist/dietician. Therefore, using and reading this guide does not establish any form of a physician-patient relationship.

Always consult with a physician or another qualified health provider with any issues or questions you might have regarding any sort of medical condition. Do not ever disregard any qualified professional medical advice or delay seeking that advice because of anything you have read in this guide. The information in this guide is not intended to be any sort of medical advice and should not be used in lieu of any medical advice by a licensed and qualified medical professional.

The information in this guide has been compiled from a variety of known sources. However, the author cannot attest to or guarantee the accuracy of each source and thus should not be held liable for any errors or omissions.

You acknowledge that the publisher of this guide will not be held liable for any loss or damage of any kind incurred as a result of this guide or the reliance on any information provided within this guide. You acknowledge and agree that you assume all risk and responsibility for any action you undertake in response to the information in this guide.

Using this guide does not guarantee any particular result (e.g., weight loss or a cure). By reading this guide, you acknowledge that there are no guarantees to any specific outcome or results you can expect.

All product names, diet plans, or names used in this guide are for identification purposes only and are the property of their respective owners. The use of these names does not imply endorsement. All other trademarks cited herein are the property of their respective owners.

Where applicable, this guide is not intended to be a substitute for the original work of this diet plan and is, at most, a supplement to the original work for this diet plan and never a direct substitute. This guide is a personal expression of the facts of that diet plan.

Where applicable, persons shown in the cover images are stock photography models and the publisher has obtained the rights to use the images through license agreements with third-party stock image companies.

Table of Contents

Introduction   7
What Is Hemochromatosis?   9
    Understanding Iron Overload and Its Symptoms   9
    Why Diet Matters in Managing Hemochromatosis   12
    Types of Hemochromatosis   13
    How Iron Is Absorbed in the Body   14
    The Role of Ferritin and Transferrin   15
Nutrition & Iron: What to Know   17
    Heme vs. Non-Heme Iron   17
    Foods That Increase Iron Absorption   19
    Nutrients That Help Inhibit Iron Absorption   20
What to Eat & What to Avoid   24
    Iron-Rich Foods to Limit or Avoid   24
    Helpful Ingredients to Incorporate   26
    Sample Grocery List & Swaps   28
Setting Up for Success   31
    Tips for Cooking Low-Iron Meals   31
    Label Reading & Meal Prep Basics   33
    Dining Out with Hemochromatosis   35
4-Week Meal Plan   37
    Week 1 Overview: Adjusting to a Low-Iron Diet & Supporting Digestion   37
    Week 2: Reducing Inflammation & Improving Energy Levels   42
    Week 3: Refining Your Diet & Maintaining Consistency   49
    Week 4: Sustaining Habits & Improving Overall Well-Being   54
Low-Iron Recipes Made Easy   60
    Energizing Breakfasts   61
    Almond Butter & Banana Smoothie Bowl   61

Quinoa Breakfast Porridge	62
Yogurt Chia Seed Parfait	63
Nourishing Lunches	64
Chickpea & Cucumber Salad	64
Lentil & Sweet Potato Soup	65
Roasted Veggie & Quinoa Bowl	66
Tofu Stir-Fry with Brown Rice	67
Light, Iron-Smart Dinners	68
Baked Cod with Zucchini Noodles	68
Black Bean & Veggie Tacos	69
Grilled Tilapia with Sweet Potato Mash	70
Lentil & Veggie Pasta	71
Snacks & Sides	72
Cucumber & Guacamole Bites	72
Yogurt & Berry Dip	73
Roasted Chickpeas	74
Hummus with Veggie Sticks	75
Refreshing Drinks & Teas	76
Iced Green Tea with Mint	76
Lemon Ginger Water	77
Berry Herbal Tea	78
Cucumber & Lime Sparkling Water	79
Lifestyle Tips for Better Management	**80**
Physical Activity and Fatigue	80
Stress, Sleep, and Iron Regulation	85
When to Talk to Your Doctor	90
Conclusion	**93**
Frequently Asked Questions (FAQs)	**96**
References and Helpful Links	**100**

Introduction

Managing hemochromatosis goes beyond simply understanding the condition; it involves adopting daily habits that help reduce its symptoms and long-term health effects. At the heart of managing this iron overload disorder is diet. What you eat plays a major role in controlling iron levels in the body, but don't worry – this doesn't mean sacrificing variety or enjoyment in your meals. By making informed food choices and following a structured approach, you can take control of your health while savoring meals that are both nourishing and delicious.

In this guide, we will talk about the following:

- All About Hemochromatosis
- Nutrition & Iron: What to Know
- What to Eat & What to Avoid
- Tips for Cooking Low-Iron Meals
- 4-Week Meal Plan
- Low-Iron Recipes Made Easy
- Lifestyle Tips for Better Management

Keep reading to learn more about managing hemochromatosis through diet and lifestyle changes. By the end, you will have a better understanding of how to make small changes to your daily routine that can have a big impact on your overall health and well-being.

What Is Hemochromatosis?

Hemochromatosis is a medical condition characterized by the body absorbing and storing excessive amounts of iron from food. Normally, the digestive process regulates iron absorption, taking in only what the body needs.

However, individuals with hemochromatosis lack this control mechanism due to a genetic mutation, leading to continuous iron accumulation. Over time, this excess iron is deposited in critical organs such as the liver, heart, and pancreas, potentially causing damage and impairing their functions.

Hemochromatosis is considered one of the most common genetic disorders in individuals of Northern European descent, though it can affect people worldwide. When left untreated, it can result in long-term complications like liver disease, diabetes, and arthritis.

Understanding Iron Overload and Its Symptoms

Iron overload happens when there is too much iron in the body. Normally, your body absorbs just the right amount of iron from the food you eat to stay healthy. But when someone has iron overload, their body absorbs and stores more iron than it needs. This extra iron doesn't leave the body on its own. Instead, it builds up in the blood and tissues over time, which can cause health problems.

This process happens gradually, so in the beginning, you might not even notice anything wrong. Early on, iron levels can rise without causing any noticeable symptoms, which is why the condition is often called "silent" during these stages. However, as more and more iron builds up, it can start to affect your body's organs like the liver, heart, pancreas, joints, and skin. That's when symptoms begin to show.

Why Symptoms Take Time to Appear

The body tends to store iron slowly, so it can take years before there's enough excess to cause damage. Many people are unaware they have iron overload until it's discovered through blood tests, often ordered for other reasons. Even when symptoms do develop, they can sometimes be mild or mistaken for something else, making it hard to get diagnosed early.

Common Symptoms of Iron Overload

When extra iron starts affecting the body, a variety of symptoms may appear. Here are some of the most common ones, explained simply:

1. ***Tiredness and Weakness***: Many people with iron overload feel constantly tired, even after a full night's sleep. This happens because too much iron can affect energy levels and make the body work harder than normal.
2. ***Joint Pain and Stiffness***: People often feel pain, stiffness, or discomfort in the joints, particularly in the fingers or knees. Over time, the extra iron in the body might settle in joints, causing inflammation and even arthritis-like symptoms.
3. ***Stomach Pain or Discomfort***: Some might experience a nagging pain or ache in the stomach area. This can happen when iron builds up in the liver or digestive system.
4. ***Changes to Skin Color***: Iron deposits in the skin can cause a noticeable darkening. Skin may appear bronze, gray, or slightly ashen, which can sometimes be mistaken for a tan.
5. ***Reduced Sex Drive or Erectile Dysfunction***: For some people, iron overload affects hormone levels. This can lead to a loss of libido (sex drive) or problems with erectile function in men.
6. ***Heart Palpitations or Irregular Heartbeats***: When iron builds up in the heart, it can cause issues like irregular heart rhythms or a fluttering feeling in the chest. Over time, this may even lead to heart-related illnesses like heart failure if untreated.

Iron overload can cause serious complications like liver damage, diabetes, or heart failure if left untreated. Symptoms such as fatigue or joint pain can be mistaken for other conditions, making proper testing, like ferritin and transferrin saturation levels, essential. Early detection and management through diet, blood donations, or medical treatments can help prevent long-term damage and protect overall health.

Why Diet Matters in Managing Hemochromatosis

Diet management is one of the most effective strategies for controlling hemochromatosis. Since the disorder revolves around excess iron absorption, monitoring and adjusting food intake can significantly slow down iron accumulation.

Reducing foods rich in easily absorbed heme iron, such as red meat and organ meats, allows individuals to lower their daily iron intake. Meanwhile, structuring meals with nutrients that inhibit iron absorption (e.g., calcium, tannins, and phytates) further limits how much the body retains. Successfully managing the condition through diet minimizes the risk of damage to vital organs and enhances quality of life.

Additionally, dietary planning helps mitigate related symptoms like fatigue. By avoiding iron spikes while maintaining a nutritionally balanced diet, individuals with hemochromatosis can sustain higher energy levels and support overall health.

Types of Hemochromatosis

There are several types of hemochromatosis, each with unique causes and presentations:

1. *Hereditary Hemochromatosis (HFE-Related)*: This is the most common form, caused by mutations in the HFE gene. Two specific mutations, C282Y and H63D, are associated with increased iron absorption. Individuals inheriting two copies (one from each parent) of the C282Y mutation are at the highest risk of developing symptoms.
2. *Secondary Hemochromatosis*: This type arises not from genetic factors but as a result of other medical conditions or treatments. Chronic blood transfusions, iron supplements, or liver diseases such as hepatitis can lead to secondary iron overload.
3. *Juvenile Hemochromatosis*: A rare, severe form of the condition that appears during adolescence or early adulthood. It is caused by mutations in genes other than HFE and results in rapid iron buildup.
4. *Neonatal Hemochromatosis*: This form affects newborns and causes severe iron overload during gestation. It is believed to be autoimmune in origin rather than genetic.
5. *Iron Loading Anemia*: Conditions such as sideroblastic anemia or thalassemia cause both anemia and iron overload. This happens because the body

raises iron absorption to compensate for the faulty blood cell production.

Understanding the specific type of hemochromatosis helps guide treatment options, ranging from dietary management to medical interventions like phlebotomy.

How Iron Is Absorbed in the Body

Iron absorption occurs primarily in the small intestine. The body tightly regulates this process under normal circumstances, absorbing only enough to meet its needs. This involves two key forms of dietary iron:

- *Heme iron*, found in animal products like meat and fish, is absorbed efficiently.
- *Non-heme iron*, found in plant-based foods, is less readily absorbed and depends on various factors, such as other nutrients present in the meal.

When the body senses low iron stores, absorption increases. When iron stores are sufficient, absorption decreases. However, in people with hemochromatosis, the mechanisms that regulate iron uptake don't function properly. This results in continued absorption regardless of iron levels already present in the body.

Other factors influencing absorption include:

- ***Enhancers***: Vitamin C and certain proteins found in meat can boost iron absorption.
- ***Inhibitors***: Compounds like calcium, tannins (found in tea and coffee), and phytates (found in whole grains and legumes) interfere with iron uptake.

By understanding how different foods and nutrients impact iron absorption, individuals with hemochromatosis can adapt their diets to reduce the risk of iron overload.

The Role of Ferritin and Transferrin

Tests to monitor iron levels are critical for diagnosing and managing hemochromatosis. Two key markers play a central role:

1. **Ferritin:**

   Ferritin is a protein that stores iron within the body's cells. Blood ferritin levels reflect how much iron is stored in the body. High ferritin levels often indicate iron overload, though levels may also rise due to inflammation or infection. Normal ferritin levels range from 24 to 336 ng/mL for men and 11 to 307 ng/mL for women.

2. **Transferrin Saturation:**

   Transferrin is a protein that transports iron in the blood. Transferrin saturation is a percentage that reflects how much of the transferrin is "loaded" with iron. A normal transferrin saturation level is below 45%. Higher percentages often point to iron overload, even before ferritin levels rise.

These markers work together to provide a comprehensive picture of iron balance. Regular monitoring of ferritin and transferrin saturation levels allows doctors to assess whether dietary changes or medical treatments are effective.

By understanding these key aspects of hemochromatosis, individuals can make informed decisions about their health. This chapter serves as the foundation for managing the condition effectively, with the next steps focusing on dietary adjustments and lifestyle strategies to limit further iron accumulation.

Nutrition & Iron: What to Know

Iron is an essential mineral that plays a critical role in overall health, particularly in producing red blood cells and supporting oxygen transport in the body. However, the way your body absorbs and processes iron depends on the type of iron in your diet and other nutrients you consume alongside it.

This chapter dives into the differences between heme and non-heme iron, explores foods that increase iron absorption, and highlights nutrients that can reduce absorption to help individuals with hemochromatosis build an iron-safe diet.

Heme vs. Non-Heme Iron

Iron from food comes in two forms, each absorbed and utilized by the body differently. Understanding these differences is key to managing iron levels.

1. **Heme Iron:**

    Heme iron comes from animal-based foods, such as meat, poultry, and fish. It gets its name because it's part of hemoglobin (the oxygen-carrying protein in blood). The body absorbs heme iron extremely efficiently, making it a significant contributor to iron levels. For people with hemochromatosis, this means reducing heme iron intake is vital to control iron overload. Foods rich in heme iron include:

- Beef, lamb, and pork
- Poultry such as chicken or turkey
- Organ meats like liver
- Seafood, including shellfish like clams and oysters

2. **Non-Heme Iron:**

Non-heme iron is found in plant-based foods, as well as in fortified or enriched products like cereal and bread. While the body doesn't absorb non-heme iron as easily, the amount absorbed depends on other factors like what else you're eating. Non-heme iron is present in:

- Leafy greens such as spinach and kale
- Legumes, including lentils, chickpeas, and beans
- Nuts and seeds
- Whole grains like oats, brown rice, and quinoa

For someone managing hemochromatosis, favoring non-heme iron sources can help reduce overall iron absorption. Additionally, knowing how to pair certain foods strategically can lower absorption further (more on this below).

Foods That Increase Iron Absorption

Some foods and nutrients can significantly enhance the body's ability to absorb iron, particularly non-heme iron. While this can be beneficial for someone with low iron levels, individuals with hemochromatosis need to be mindful of these enhancers and how they influence iron uptake.

1. **Vitamin C:**

    Vitamin C, or ascorbic acid, is one of the strongest enhancers of non-heme iron absorption. It converts iron into a form the body can absorb more easily. This means that pairing vitamin C-rich foods with iron-containing plant foods increases iron absorption significantly.

    For those managing hemochromatosis, it's better to avoid pairing these foods with meals rich in non-heme iron or opt to have vitamin C-rich snacks between meals.

    Foods high in vitamin C include:

    - Citrus fruits like oranges, lemons, and grapefruits
    - Strawberries, kiwis, and pineapples
    - Bell peppers, tomatoes, and broccoli

2. **Meat, Fish, and Poultry Factor:**

   Proteins in meat, fish, and poultry enhance the absorption of both heme and non-heme iron. This effect is often referred to as the "meat factor." Even small amounts of meat combined with plant-based dishes can boost non-heme iron absorption.

   To manage iron overload, avoiding or limiting these foods during meals can help reduce absorption.

3. **Acidic Foods:**

   Acidic foods, like vinegar or fermented foods, can enhance iron absorption as well. Using lemon juice or vinegar-based dressings on salads may increase iron uptake from plant-based ingredients.

Understanding how certain foods enhance iron absorption is crucial for managing iron levels effectively. Whether you're boosting low iron or controlling iron overload, being mindful of these dietary factors can make a significant difference.

Nutrients That Help Inhibit Iron Absorption

Thankfully, certain nutrients and compounds naturally reduce iron absorption by binding to iron or interfering with the process. Including these "inhibitors" in meals can make it easier for individuals with hemochromatosis to limit iron absorption.

1. **Calcium:**

   Calcium hinders iron absorption by competing with iron for absorption in the gut. It is effective against both heme and non-heme iron. Foods rich in calcium include:

   Including calcium-rich foods as part of meals is a simple way to slow down iron absorption.

   - Dairy products like milk, cheese, and yogurt
   - Calcium-fortified plant-based milks
   - Leafy greens such as kale and collard greens

2. **Tannins:**

   Tannins are compounds found in tea, coffee, and some herbal teas. They bind to iron, keeping it from being fully absorbed. Tannins are particularly effective at blocking non-heme iron.

   Tips for an iron-safe diet:

   - Drinking tea or coffee with meals instead of between them.
   - Choosing herbal teas with high tannin content, like black or green tea.

3. **Phytates:**

   Found in whole grains, seeds, nuts, and legumes, phytates bind to iron and reduce its bioavailability. While not enough to cause deficiency in most people, this effect can be helpful for managing high iron levels in those with hemochromatosis. Common phytate-rich foods include:

- Brown rice, oats, and whole wheat
- Almonds, walnuts, and sunflower seeds
- Beans, lentils, and chickpeas

4. **Polyphenols:**

Polyphenols are plant-based compounds with antioxidant properties, but they also interfere with iron absorption. They are found in many fruits, vegetables, herbs, and beverages like tea, coffee, and wine.

Examples include:

- Berries, apples, and plums
- Spinach, onions, and celery
- Cocoa and dark chocolate

Using these inhibitors wisely can make a big difference in reducing iron absorption from meals. For example, pairing a whole grain meal with a glass of tea or incorporating yogurt can help slow down how much iron the body absorbs.

Understanding how iron is absorbed, as well as the role of enhancers and inhibitors, allows individuals with hemochromatosis to make more informed dietary choices. Limiting heme iron sources, being cautious about vitamin C-rich food pairings, and including inhibitors like calcium-rich foods can help reduce iron overload effectively.

By paying attention to how different foods work together, people with hemochromatosis can build a balanced and enjoyable diet that supports their overall well-being and long-term health.

What to Eat & What to Avoid

Managing iron levels through diet is a key strategy for individuals living with hemochromatosis. By knowing which foods to limit or avoid, as well as which ones to include, it's possible to build a sustainable eating plan that supports long-term health.

This chapter outlines iron-rich foods to watch out for, ingredients to incorporate into your meals, and a handy grocery list with easy swaps to make your shopping simpler.

Iron-Rich Foods to Limit or Avoid

Since hemochromatosis involves excessive iron absorption, it's essential to limit foods high in iron, especially those rich in easily absorbed heme iron. Here's what to watch out for:

1. **Red Meat:**
   - Steak, beef, lamb, and pork are all heme iron-rich and contribute significantly to iron buildup.
   - Reduce your intake of these meats, or only eat them in small portions.

2. **Organ Meats:**
   - Liver, kidney, and other organ meats contain extremely high amounts of heme iron.
   - These should be avoided almost entirely if you're managing iron overload.
3. **Shellfish:**
   - Clams, mussels, and oysters provide substantial amounts of heme iron.
   - Opt for plant-based alternatives or non-heme iron protein sources instead.
4. **Iron-Fortified Foods:**
   - Breakfast cereals, breads, and pasta often have added iron, which isn't ideal for those with hemochromatosis.
   - Look for non-fortified options on labels to avoid unnecessary iron.
5. **Alcohol (in Excess):**
   - Alcohol, particularly red wine, can exacerbate iron absorption and increase the risk of liver damage.
   - Limit alcohol to moderate or occasional consumption if your doctor allows it.
6. **Vitamin C with High-Iron Meals:**
   - While vitamin C is healthy, pairing it with iron-rich foods boosts iron absorption.

- Avoid combining foods like oranges, bell peppers, or tomatoes with meals heavy in non-heme iron (such as lentils or spinach).

Managing hemochromatosis requires being mindful of iron-rich foods and making dietary adjustments to reduce iron absorption. By limiting heme iron sources and avoiding certain combinations, you can help protect your health and manage iron levels effectively.

Helpful Ingredients to Incorporate

While some foods should be limited, there are many others that can actively help reduce iron absorption or enhance nutrient balance. Including these ingredients in your diet can make managing iron overload simpler and more enjoyable:

1. **Calcium-Rich Foods:**
   - Dairy products like milk, cheese, and yogurt block iron absorption when consumed with meals.
   - Fortified plant-based milks, such as almond or oat milk, are great alternatives if you're avoiding dairy.
2. **Whole Grains:**
   - Brown rice, quinoa, oats, and barley contain phytates, which reduce iron absorption.
   - They are also nutrient-dense and support overall health.

3. **Nuts and Seeds:**
   - Almonds, walnuts, sunflower seeds, and chia seeds are not only rich in healthy fats but also contain phytates that inhibit iron uptake.
4. **Legumes and Lentils:**
   - Chickpeas, lentils, and black beans provide protein without contributing significantly to iron overload, especially when paired with calcium sources.
5. **Tea and Coffee:**
   - Both contain tannins, which reduce iron absorption if consumed with meals.
   - Incorporate these beverages into your routine as a simple strategy to lower iron levels.
6. **Fruits and Vegetables (Away from Iron-Rich Meals):**
   - While vitamin C-rich foods enhance iron absorption, enjoying them as snacks or separate meals gives you the benefits while minimizing risk.
   - Berries, apples, cucumbers, and leafy greens are excellent choices.

Incorporating these ingredients into your diet can help manage iron overload while supporting overall health. With simple adjustments, you can balance nutrients and enjoy a variety of delicious, nutrient-dense foods.

Sample Grocery List & Swaps

Here's a practical list of foods you can include in your shopping, along with beneficial swaps to replace high-iron or iron-enhancing items:

1. **Fruits & Vegetables:**
     - Apples, berries, and grapes (swap for citrus fruits with iron-rich meals).
     - Cucumbers, zucchini, and celery.
     - Leafy greens like lettuce or arugula (instead of spinach or kale at mealtime).
     - Onions, leeks, and eggplants.
2. **Proteins:**
     - Buy: Legumes (lentils, chickpeas, black beans), tofu, and eggs (as a moderate-histidine option).
     - Swap: Red meat and seafood for plant-based protein sources.
3. **Grains & Breads:**
     - Buy: Oats, quinoa, barley, and groceries labeled "whole grain."
     - Swap: Iron-fortified cereals and white pasta for non-enriched options like buckwheat noodles or whole wheat tortillas.
4. **Dairy Products:**
     - Milk, yogurt, and cheese (or dairy substitutes like fortified almond, soy, or cashew milk).

5. **Snacks & Add-ons:**
    - Almonds, walnuts, sunflower seeds, and chia seeds.
    - Unsweetened tea (green or black), coffee, and herbal tea options for after meals.
    - Dark chocolate with a high cocoa content (over 70%).
6. **Condiments & Cooking Staples:**
    - Olive oil, vinegar, or mustard for dressings.
    - Avoid high-acidity items like excessive tomato-based sauces when paired with iron-rich meals.

Easy Swaps in Action

- Instead of a steak salad topped with oranges and a side of beer, opt for a quinoa salad with almonds, arugula, and a light vinegar dressing. Pair it with a refreshing cup of tea.
- Swap fortified cereals with calcium-rich yogurt topped with berries and chia seeds for breakfast.
- Replace spaghetti Bolognese with a whole-grain pasta tossed in olive oil, steamed vegetables, and a sprinkle of parmesan.

By focusing on these suggested foods and swapping high-iron options for safer alternatives, individuals managing hemochromatosis can enjoy a varied and satisfying diet while protecting their health. Keep experimenting with new recipes and combinations to keep meals enjoyable while staying on track!

Setting Up for Success

Managing hemochromatosis can feel overwhelming at first, but with a few adjustments, you can set yourself up for success. This chapter focuses on practical ways to make cooking, grocery shopping, and dining out easier while managing iron levels. Whether you're in your kitchen or at a restaurant, the tips below will help you stay on track without sacrificing flavor or enjoyment.

Tips for Cooking Low-Iron Meals

Cooking at home allows you to control what goes into your meals, making it one of the best ways to manage iron intake. Here are some tips to prepare delicious, low-iron meals that fit your lifestyle:

1. **Choose the Right Ingredients:**
    - Focus on non-heme iron sources like legumes, nuts, seeds, and whole grains instead of red meat or organ meats.

- Incorporate calcium-rich foods such as dairy products or fortified plant-based milks to naturally reduce iron absorption.

2. **Pair Foods Wisely:**
   - Avoid combining high-iron foods with Vitamin C-rich ingredients (like citrus fruits, bell peppers, or tomatoes), as Vitamin C boosts iron absorption.
   - Use inhibitors like tea, coffee, or dairy during or immediately after meals to help limit iron uptake.

3. **Try Acidic Alternatives:**

   Swap out vinegar and acidic marinades when cooking iron-heavy meals, as acidic ingredients can enhance absorption. Use herbs, olive oil, and low-acidity seasonings instead.

4. **Experiment with Spices and Herbs:**

   Add flavor with spices such as turmeric, garlic, ginger, and basil instead of relying on iron-rich condiments or meat-based broths.

5. **Plan Balanced Meals:**

   Include plenty of fresh vegetables, whole grains, and plant-based proteins to create nutrient-dense but iron-conscious meals. A stir fry with tofu and broccoli over brown rice is a great everyday dinner option.

6. **Cook in Non-Iron Utensils:**

   Avoid cooking in cast-iron pots and pans, as this can add extra iron to your food. Use stainless steel, glass, or ceramic cookware instead.

By making mindful ingredient choices and cooking techniques, you can create flavorful, low-iron meals that support your health goals. With a bit of planning, it's easy to enjoy nutritious dishes tailored to your needs.

Label Reading & Meal Prep Basics

Navigating grocery stores and preparing meals at home becomes much easier when you know what to look for. Here's how to simplify the process:

1. **Read Food Labels Carefully:**
   - Watch for labels on cereals, breads, and other fortified products that list added iron. Opt for non-fortified or wholefood alternatives instead.
   - Check the ingredient list for words like "iron-fortified" or "ferrous sulfate."
2. **Understand Serving Sizes:**

   Keep serving sizes in mind, especially for foods like meat or iron-rich snacks. Stick to small portions if you're including these in your meals.

3. **Create a Weekly Meal Plan:**
   - Map out your meals for the week, making sure to include foods that inhibit absorption, such as dairy, whole grains, and legumes.
   - Prep ingredients ahead of time to save effort during busy weekdays. For example, cook a big batch of quinoa or lentils to use in salads, soups, or side dishes throughout the week.

4. **Practice Portion Control:**

   Balance iron intake by combining iron-rich foods with iron inhibitors. For instance, if you have a meal with spinach or legumes, pair it with a dairy-based dressing or tea.

5. **Stock Your Pantry:**

   Keep staple ingredients like oats, nuts, beans, rice, non-fortified cereals, and herb seasonings on hand. A well-stocked pantry makes it easier to throw together quick, iron-conscious meals.

6. **Freeze What You Don't Use:**

   To avoid waste, freeze extras in meal-sized portions. Soups, stews, cooked beans, and grains are all freezer-friendly, making future meal prep quick and hassle-free.

Mastering label reading and meal prep can make healthy eating more manageable and stress-free. With a little planning and the right pantry staples, you can create balanced, iron-conscious meals that fit your lifestyle.

Dining Out with Hemochromatosis

Enjoying meals at restaurants or social gatherings is possible with a little preparation. Use these strategies to make eating out a stress-free experience:

1. **Research Menus Ahead of Time**: Check restaurant menus online in advance and choose meals with vegetables, whole grains, and lean proteins. Avoid dishes with red or organ meats like steak or liver.
2. **Ask Questions**: Don't hesitate to ask your server about how dishes are prepared. Questions like "Does this contain fortified grains?" or "Does this include red meat or organ meat?" can help you avoid unexpected iron-rich ingredients.
3. **Customize Your Meal**: Request modifications to suit your needs. For example, ask for dressings or sauces on the side to reduce vitamin C exposure or swap red meat for extra vegetables. Many restaurants are happy to make adjustments if you explain your dietary needs.
4. **Watch Out for Hidden Sources of Iron**: Be cautious of iron-rich extras like shellfish-based soups, fortified pasta, or cooked spinach. Opt for alternatives like vegetable-based soups or salads with non-iron-heavy toppings.

5. ***Drink Smart***: Pair your meal with beverages that inhibit iron absorption, such as tea, coffee, or milk. Avoid pairing wine, juice, or cocktails with high-iron meals as these can enhance absorption.
6. ***Portion Out Leftovers***: Restaurant portions are often large. Consider splitting a meal with a friend or taking half of it home to maintain portion control.

By following these practical tips and staying proactive, you'll find it easier to maintain an iron-safe lifestyle at home and wherever you go. Taking small but consistent steps toward managing your meals can greatly reduce the risk of iron overload while keeping life fun, flavorful, and free from unnecessary worry.

4-Week Meal Plan

Managing hemochromatosis requires careful planning, but it doesn't have to be complicated. This 4-week meal plan is focused on maintaining energy, reducing symptoms, and avoiding excess iron accumulation. Each week has a specific focus to help you stay on track while keeping meals enjoyable and manageable. You'll also find meal prep tips to make your cooking routine more efficient.

Week 1 Overview: Adjusting to a Low-Iron Diet & Supporting Digestion

Starting a low-iron diet can feel overwhelming, but Week 1 is all about gradually adjusting your eating habits to reduce iron intake without sacrificing flavor or nutrition. This phase eases you into new routines with a focus on whole grains, fresh vegetables, and lean or plant-based proteins.

It also emphasizes avoiding iron-rich foods like red meat, organ meats, and iron-fortified products to prevent iron overload. At the same time, we'll include foods that promote digestion to keep your energy levels balanced and your body feeling supported.

Daily Breakdown

Days 1-3: Replace Red Meat and Organ Meats

Your first three days will focus on phasing out high-heme iron foods like red meat (beef, lamb) and organ meats (liver, kidneys) while replacing them with lower-iron protein options like chicken, fish, and plant-based alternatives. Whole grains and lightly cooked vegetables will round out your meals.

Example Meals for Days 1-3:

- *Breakfast*: Overnight oats made with almond milk, chia seeds, and fresh berries. Avoid adding iron-fortified oatmeal.
- *Lunch*: Grilled chicken salad with mixed greens, cherry tomatoes, cucumber, and feta cheese, dressed with olive oil and lemon. Serve with a side of quinoa.
- *Dinner*: Pan-seared cod with garlic and lemon, served alongside steamed broccoli and roasted sweet potatoes.
- *Snacks*: Carrot sticks with hummus, apple slices with a small handful of walnuts, or Greek yogurt with a drizzle of honey.

Tips:

- Start shifting your protein choices away from red meat by preparing chicken or fish in simple ways, like grilling or baking, with light seasonings.

- Enhance digestion by including fibrous foods like vegetables and whole grains in every meal.

Days 4-5: Add Salads and Dairy for Iron Blocking

Focus on incorporating more leafy greens, fresh salads, and dairy products to help inhibit iron absorption. Pairing meals with dairy, such as milk, cheese, or yogurt, reduces non-heme iron absorption from plant-based foods. Cut out sugary snacks and processed foods that can irritate digestion and spike blood sugar levels.

Example Meals for Days 4-5:

- *Breakfast*: Smoothie made with spinach, banana, Greek yogurt, and unsweetened almond milk. Add a pinch of cinnamon for flavor.
- *Lunch*: Lentil salad with arugula, diced cucumber, red onion, and a dollop of plain yogurt as a dressing.
- *Dinner*: Zucchini noodles (or whole-grain pasta) with a garlic cream sauce, topped with sautéed bell peppers and mushrooms. Grate parmesan cheese over the top to enhance flavor and block iron absorption.
- *Snacks*: Hard-boiled eggs, whole-grain crackers with ricotta cheese, or celery sticks with almond butter.

Tips:

- Pair greens like arugula or spinach with a calcium-rich food, like cheese, to limit iron absorption.

- Since cooking reduces the oxalates in some vegetables (which naturally inhibit iron), balance raw and cooked greens throughout your week.

Days 6-7: Experiment with Low-Iron Recipes

Wrap up the week by trying simple low-iron recipes that are satisfying and nutrient-dense. Use ingredients like legumes, lentils, and root vegetables. Pair these with teas or coffee during meals; the tannins in these beverages help reduce iron absorption further.

Example Meals for Days 6-7:

- *Breakfast*: Savory oatmeal bowl topped with sautéed mushrooms, a soft-boiled egg, and a sprinkle of cheese.
- *Lunch*: A vegetable soup made with carrots, celery, potatoes, and a handful of lentils, paired with whole-grain bread.
- *Dinner*: Stir-fried tofu with bok choy, bell peppers, sesame oil, and a splash of soy sauce. Serve over brown rice.
- *Snacks*: A small handful of roasted almonds, unsweetened yogurt with diced mango, or cucumber slices with a squeeze of lemon juice.

Tips:

- Experiment with spice blends to keep meals exciting while avoiding processed marinades, which often contain hidden sugars or iron fortifications.
- Brew a large batch of herbal iced tea (like peppermint or chamomile) to drink with meals throughout the week, as these can help inhibit iron absorption while keeping you hydrated.

Meal Prep Tips for Week 1

To stay on track and simplify your week, strategize your meal prep. Proper preparation ensures that healthier low-iron options are always available, reducing the temptation to default to high-iron foods:

1. **Batch Cooking Grains**: Cook several cups of quinoa, rice, or farro at the start of the week. Store in airtight containers in the fridge, so they're ready to use in salads, bowls, or as sides for meals.
2. **Prepping Vegetables**: Wash, peel, and chop vegetables in advance. Store them in separate containers to maintain freshness. These can be added to salads, roasted, or sautéed as needed.
3. **Make Your Own Condiments**: To control hidden ingredients, prepare simple dressings or dips at home. Examples include tahini-lemon dressing, plain yogurt-based dips, and olive oil with fresh herbs.

4. ***Prepare Snacks in Bulk***: Portion out servings of nuts, veggie sticks, or hard-boiled eggs into grab-and-go containers to avoid processed snacks.
5. ***Freezer-Friendly Options***: Make a large pot of soup or stew and freeze individual portions. This ensures you have an easy, nutrient-rich meal on hand when you don't have time to cook.

Pro-Tip for Beginners:

Keep a food diary this week to note how your body reacts to the dietary changes. Tracking meals, symptoms, and energy levels can help you stay mindful and spot connections, such as which foods make you feel better or worse.

By the end of Week 1, you should feel more comfortable with the basics of a low-iron diet and confident in preparing balanced, nourishing meals. Use what you've learned to build momentum for the following weeks!

Week 2: Reducing Inflammation & Improving Energy Levels

Week 2 builds on the success of Week 1 by introducing more anti-inflammatory foods and fine-tuning nutrient-dense options that help ease symptoms like joint pain and fatigue. This week also reinforces the principles of a low-iron diet while expanding meal variety. With vibrant, colorful ingredients and energizing options like fatty fish, whole grains, and nuts, you'll sustain momentum toward better health.

For anyone transitioning from Week 1 to Week 2, the groundwork you've laid in identifying low-iron meals and balanced combinations will make this week's changes smoother. The goal for these seven days is to reduce discomfort while fueling your body with sustainable energy.

Daily Breakdown

Day 8-9: Add Omega-3 Fats and Vibrant Veggies

Start the week by introducing fatty fish such as salmon or mackerel for their rich Omega-3 content. These healthy fats help combat inflammation. Pair them with colorful vegetables like zucchini, cauliflower, and carrots to fill your meals with antioxidants and fiber.

Example Meals:

- ***Breakfast***: Scrambled eggs cooked in olive oil, served with arugula and avocado slices on the side. Add a whole-grain toast.
- ***Lunch***: Grilled salmon salad with mixed greens, roasted cherry tomatoes, cucumbers, and balsamic vinaigrette.
- ***Dinner***: Baked mackerel with a side of roasted sweet potatoes and steamed broccoli.

- *Snacks*: Bell pepper slices with hummus, a handful of walnuts, or plain Greek yogurt topped with blueberries.

Tips:

- Roast salmon or mackerel in advance for quick meal prep. Season with garlic and herbs for added flavor.
- Keep pre-cut vegetables in your fridge to easily stir-fry or roast later.

Day 10: Focus on Anti-Inflammatory Spices & Whole Grains

Introduce spices like turmeric, ginger, and cinnamon to further reduce inflammation. Pair these with whole grains, such as barley or bulgur, for meals that are both hearty and nutrient-dense.

Example Meals:

- *Breakfast*: Porridge made with bulgur, almond milk, cinnamon, and apple slices.
- *Lunch*: Barley salad with grilled zucchini, fresh parsley, and a drizzle of tahini-lemon dressing. Add a boiled egg for protein.
- *Dinner*: Curried sweet potato and lentil stew spiced with turmeric and cumin. Serve with a side of steamed green beans.

- *Snacks*: Sliced mango with a sprinkle of chili powder, almonds, or herbal tea with a piece of dark chocolate (70% cocoa or higher).

Tips:

- Make a large batch of barley or bulgur early in the week to save time. Use as a base for fresh salads or warm bowls.
- Pre-mix spice blends for stews or roasted vegetables to simplify cooking.

Day 11-12: Brighten Meals with Fermented Foods & Intensify Variety

Fermented foods like yogurt and sauerkraut are excellent for gut health, while brightly colored vegetables like bell peppers and greens keep inflammation down. These days emphasize variety and vibrant flavors to keep meals exciting.

Example Meals:

- *Breakfast*: Smoothie bowl blended with spinach, frozen berries, almond milk, and chia seeds. Top with granola or sunflower seeds.
- *Lunch*: Roasted vegetable bowl with farro, sautéed kale, and a dollop of yogurt-tahini sauce. Add sauerkraut on the side.

- **Dinner**: Herb-crusted baked trout with roasted Brussels sprouts and mashed carrots. Finish with freshly squeezed lemon.
- **Snacks**: Cucumber slices with tzatziki, rice cakes with almond butter, or kefir with a drizzle of honey.

Tips:

- Pre-roast vegetable trays to reduce cooking time during busy workdays.
- Incorporate sauerkraut or kimchi into salads or bowls for an added probiotic punch.

Day 13: Hydrate & Reset Using Simple, Fresh Ingredients

Include hydrating foods like cucumbers, watermelon, or greens to refresh your system. Simplicity is key as you wind down the week, prioritizing fresh, vibrant ingredients.

Example Meals:

- **Breakfast**: Overnight oats layered with coconut yogurt, blueberries, and a sprinkling of chia seeds.
- **Lunch**: Mixed green salad with shredded carrots, bell peppers, soft-boiled egg, and avocado. Drizzle with olive oil and balsamic vinegar.
- **Dinner**: Grilled chicken breast with roasted zucchini and a quinoa pilaf. End with a cup of herbal tea.
- **Snacks**: Fresh watermelon slices, carrot sticks with hummus, or snap peas.

Tips:

- Chop and store fruits, like watermelon and cantaloupe, in advance for an instant hydrating snack.
- Plan meals with minimal prep time to reduce stress and enjoy fresh flavors.

Day 14: Review, Reflect, and Transition to Week 3

Wrap up the week by reviewing your progress, refining your routine, and using what you've learned to plan ahead. Revisit favorite meals from Week 2 and enjoy a mix of protein, whole grains, and colorful vegetables to end the week strong.

Example Meals:

- *Breakfast*: Sautéed spinach and scrambled eggs with a side of fresh berries and toast.
- *Lunch*: Quinoa bowl with roasted sweet potatoes, chickpeas, kale, and tahini dressing. Top with a sprinkle of sesame seeds.
- *Dinner*: Grilled salmon served with mashed cauliflower and steamed asparagus. Add fresh herbs for extra flavor.
- *Snacks*: A handful of trail mix, orange slices, or herbal tea with whole-grain crackers topped with ricotta cheese.

Tips:

- Freeze leftover fish or roasted veggies in portioned containers for quick meals in Week 3.
- Take notes on standout recipes or ingredients that made you feel energized and include them in future meal plans.

Meal Prep Tips for Week 2

1. **Cook Proteins in Advance**: Marinate and bake or grill fish, chicken, or tofu at the start of the week. Store in airtight containers for easy reheating.
2. **Batch Roast Veggies**: Prepare large trays of roasted broccoli, Brussels sprouts, zucchini, or sweet potatoes to use as sides.
3. **Pre-Blend Smoothie Packs**: Freeze pre-portioned fruits and greens in resealable bags so you can quickly blend with almond milk or yogurt.
4. **Double Soups & Stews**: Make large portions of lentil soup or sweet potato curry and freeze extra servings for stress-free meals.
5. **Snack Prep**: Divide nuts, seeds, or carrot sticks into small containers to avoid relying on processed options.

Pro-Tip for Week 2:

Track your energy levels and digestion throughout the week. This will help you discover which meals are fueling your body best, giving you the insight to sustain these changes in Week 3 and beyond.

By the end of Week 2, you'll notice reduced inflammation, improved energy, and greater confidence in maintaining a low-iron lifestyle. You're now fully prepared to transition into Week 3, focusing on balance and sustainability.

Week 3: Refining Your Diet & Maintaining Consistency

Week 3 is an opportunity to refine your low-iron meal plan while expanding variety and maintaining consistency in your routine. You'll build on the momentum from Weeks 1 and 2 by diversifying your meals, incorporating more legumes, nuts, and fermented foods, and finding new ways to sustain energy levels throughout the day. This week focuses on balance, creativity, and small dietary adjustments that make low-iron eating enjoyable and sustainable for the long term.

With your foundation set, Week 3 encourages you to deepen your knowledge of ingredient pairings, keep meals interesting, and streamline your prep strategies for easy adherence.

Daily Breakdown

Day 15-16: Incorporate Whole-Grain Pasta or Couscous

Kick off the week by preparing simple, comforting meals featuring whole-grain pasta or couscous. Use light, veggie-based sauces and add a calcium source like grated parmesan or yogurt to further inhibit iron absorption.

Example Meals:

- ***Breakfast***: Savory oatmeal made with almond milk, spinach, and a poached egg, topped with a sprinkle of feta cheese.
- ***Lunch***: Whole-grain couscous bowl with roasted zucchini, chickpeas, cherry tomatoes, and hummus. Add a side of plain yogurt with a drizzle of olive oil and herbs for dipping.
- ***Dinner***: Pasta primavera with whole-grain noodles, sautéed bell peppers, carrots, and mushrooms in a light olive oil and garlic sauce. Sprinkle with grated parmesan.
- ***Snacks***: Whole-grain crackers with cream cheese, apple slices with almond butter, or roasted nuts.

Tips:

- Cook extra pasta or couscous for lunches and dinners later in the week.
- Store leftover veggie sauces in small containers to use as convenient add-ons to other dishes.

Day 17-19: Explore Vegetarian Recipes with Legumes and Nuts

This midweek stretch highlights vegetarian recipes featuring legumes like lentils, chickpeas, and kidney beans. Pair these with calcium sources like cheese, yogurt, or tahini-based dressings to limit iron absorption without sacrificing protein.

Example Meals:

- **_Breakfast_**: Yogurt parfait layered with granola, sliced bananas, and chia seeds.
- **_Lunch_**: Lentil and vegetable curry served with brown rice or quinoa, paired with a dollop of yogurt for balance.
- **_Dinner_**: Chickpea and spinach stew cooked with garlic, fresh parsley, and a touch of coconut milk, served with whole-grain flatbread.
- **_Snacks_**: Sliced cucumbers with tahini dip, a handful of walnuts, or fresh orange segments.

Tips:

- Pre-soak or pre-cook legumes over the weekend to make quick meals during busy weekdays.
- Experiment with plant-based recipes by incorporating spices like cumin, coriander, and paprika to intensify flavor.

Day 20-21: Introduce Fermented Foods & Fresh Herbs

Wrap up Week 3 by prioritizing gut health with fermented foods like yogurt or kefir, alongside fresh herbs like parsley, cilantro, or dill for added vibrancy and flavor. These days help you reconnect with lighter, nutrient-rich meals after the hearty legumes and grains earlier in the week.

Example Meals:

- **Breakfast**: Smoothie made with kefir, frozen berries, spinach, and a handful of avocado.
- **Lunch**: Herb-packed quinoa salad with fresh parsley, chopped cucumbers, diced tomatoes, and a yogurt-lemon dressing. Add roasted chicken for extra protein if desired.
- **Dinner**: Salmon and roasted vegetable bowl with a side of sauerkraut or kimchi, dressed with tahini and fresh cilantro for garnish.
- **Snacks**: Plain kefir with a drizzle of honey, unsalted sunflower seeds, or celery sticks dipped in guacamole.

Tips:

- Pre-chop fresh herbs and store them in airtight bags or containers to sprinkle onto meals easily.
- Blend plain kefir or yogurt with fruit and greens to make refreshing, probiotic-rich smoothies.

Meal Prep Tips for Week 3

1. **Batch-Cook Soups or Stews**: Prepare large portions of lentil curry, chickpea stew, or vegetable soup to freeze in individual servings for later use.
2. **Pre-Soak or Cook Legumes**: Cut down prep time by soaking beans like chickpeas or lentils overnight or cooking them in advance and storing in the refrigerator.

3. **Pre-Make Yogurt Parfaits**: Create parfaits in mason jars using granola, fruits, and yogurt for quick, grab-and-go breakfasts or snacks.
4. **Double Sauces or Dressings**: Make extra light veggie-based pasta sauces, yogurt dressings, or tahini dips to pair with proteins and grains throughout the week.
5. **Snack Packs**: Divide nuts, seeds, or roasted chickpeas into small portions to make healthy snacking easier.

Pro-Tip for Week 3:

Track how the new ingredients and meal combinations make you feel. Does incorporating fermented foods improve digestion? Do you feel more energized with lentil-based meals? Reflect on these insights to personalize your plan as you prepare for Week 4.

By the end of Week 3, you'll have polished your low-iron diet routine, tried interesting new recipes, and built confidence in meal prep strategies. With improved gut health, consistent energy, and a wide variety of meals, you'll be ready to round out your plan with Week 4's focus on long-term sustainability and lifestyle integration.

Week 4: Sustaining Habits & Improving Overall Well-Being

This final week focuses on strengthening the habits you've developed over the past three weeks. It's about consistency, mindful eating, and finding flexibility within your low-iron framework. By revisiting favorite meals, staying hydrated, and refining your routines, you'll be setting yourself up for long-term success. Think of this week as an opportunity to fine-tune your diet while prioritizing both balance and enjoyment.

Let's take these final seven days step-by-step to ensure you finish this plan with confidence and energy.

Daily Breakdown

Day 22-23: Hydrate and Replenish

Hydration takes center stage as you integrate herbal teas and water-rich foods into your day. Pair meals with non-heme iron sources like vegetables and nuts, while continuing to focus on a diverse plate.

Example Meals:

- ***Breakfast***: Oatmeal cooked with almond milk, topped with blueberries, sliced almonds, and a drizzle of honey.

- *Lunch*: Spinach and lentil salad with roasted beets, walnuts, and a light lemon vinaigrette. Drink a cup of chamomile tea.
- *Dinner*: Baked cod with steamed broccoli, mashed sweet potatoes, and a side of arugula salad. Pair with peppermint tea to support digestion.
- *Snacks*: Fresh celery sticks with hummus, orange slices, or a small handful of walnuts.

Tips:

- Use an herbal tea or water infusion (like cucumber or mint water) to replace sugary or caffeinated beverages.
- Prep salads in jars or containers the night before to make lunch stress-free.

Day 24-25: Revisit and Customize Favorite Recipes

Continue with your trusted meals but modify them for variety. Swap ingredients, explore new spices, or redesign dishes with seasonal produce to keep meals interesting.

Example Meals:

- *Breakfast*: Greek yogurt topped with granola, peach slices, and chia seeds.
- *Lunch*: Chickpea and roasted red pepper pasta made with whole-grain penne, dressed with olive oil and fresh basil.

- **Dinner**: Stir-fried tofu with bell peppers, broccoli, and a light sesame-soy glaze, served over barley.
- **Snacks**: Roasted unsalted sunflower seeds, cucumber slices with tzatziki, or fresh melon cubes.

Tips:

- Repurpose leftovers by mixing them into wraps, grain bowls, or salads.
- Play with fresh herbs like dill, basil, or cilantro to brighten your favorite dishes.

Day 26-27: Flexibility and Flavor Exploration

Allow flexibility by incorporating meals that align with cravings while staying within a healthy framework. Focus on nutrient balance and portion control when indulging in comfort dishes.

Example Meals:

- **Breakfast**: Savory French toast made from whole-grain bread, paired with sautéed spinach and a poached egg.
- **Lunch**: Veggie-packed quesadillas featuring black beans, diced peppers, and mozzarella cheese. Serve with a spinach, avocado, and tomato salad.
- **Dinner**: Grilled chicken and vegetable kabobs, served over quinoa with a dollop of yogurt-based herb sauce.

- *Snacks*: Kefir mixed with frozen berries, roasted almonds with a dusting of cinnamon, or homemade veggie chips.

Tips:

- When craving food that feels indulgent, balance heavier dishes with light, fresh sides.
- Try cooking something new, like swapping chicken for baked tofu or experimenting with fun pasta shapes.

Day 28: Reflection and Moving Forward

Your final day is all about reflecting on what worked while enjoying the meals you've come to love. Create balance with simple, nourishing dishes that allow you to close the week feeling accomplished.

Example Meals:

- *Breakfast*: Quinoa porridge topped with dried cranberries, chopped pecans, and a drizzle of maple syrup.
- *Lunch*: Grilled salmon salad with mixed greens, roasted sweet potatoes, and a yogurt-lemon dressing.
- *Dinner*: Lentil soup with a side of whole-grain flatbread and a refreshing tomato-cucumber salad. Finish with a light herbal tea.

- ***Snacks***: Small handful of trail mix, apple slices with almond butter, or whole-grain crackers paired with ricotta and chopped parsley.

Tips:

- Think about adapting your plan beyond the 4 weeks by identifying quick, go-to meals.
- Start brainstorming more on-the-go options or seasonal twists to adjust your menu throughout the year.

Meal Prep Tips for Week 4

1. ***Plan a Flexible Menu***: Combine favorite recipes from past weeks with new ideas or crave-worthy dishes.
2. ***Create a Hydration Routine***: Make herbal teas or infused waters a part of your daily habits.
3. ***Stock Freezer Staples***: Items like soups, roasted vegetables, and pre-cooked grains can be stored for easy meal prep.
4. ***Pre-Portion Snacks***: Divide your snacks into grab-and-go servings to stay prepared and avoid impulse eating.
5. ***Rotate Ingredients***: Keep meals exciting by alternating between different veggies, proteins, and grains.

Pro-Tip for Week 4:

Set time aside each week to reflect on your favorite meals and how they've impacted your overall well-being. Use this insight to build a lasting, enjoyable meal plan going forward.

Across these four weeks, you've learned how to manage your hemochromatosis with a low-iron, nutrient-dense diet. Week by week, you've balanced practicality with progress, creating a sustainable approach to eating that prioritizes your health. With a focus on hydration, flexibility, and mindful choices, Week 4 ensures you finish empowered to confidently maintain these habits long-term.

Low-Iron Recipes Made Easy

Managing hemochromatosis doesn't mean giving up on delicious and satisfying meals. Below you'll find a collection of easy, low-iron recipes that cater to every part of your day. These options are designed to keep your energy up while managing iron levels effectively.

Energizing Breakfasts

Almond Butter & Banana Smoothie Bowl

Ingredients:

- 1 frozen banana
- 1 cup almond milk
- 2 tablespoons almond butter
- 1 teaspoon chia seeds
- 5–6 fresh berries (for topping)
- 2 tablespoons granola (non-fortified)

Instructions:

1. In a blender, combine the frozen banana, almond milk, almond butter, and chia seeds.
2. Blend until smooth and creamy.
3. Pour into a bowl and top with fresh berries and granola.
4. Enjoy your iron-rich and delicious breakfast!

Quinoa Breakfast Porridge

Ingredients:

- 1/3 cup cooked quinoa
- 1 cup almond milk
- 1 tablespoon maple syrup
- 1/4 teaspoon cinnamon
- 1 tablespoon chopped almonds

Instructions:

1. In a small saucepan, combine the cooked quinoa and almond milk.
2. Cook over medium heat until it starts to simmer.
3. Stir in the maple syrup and cinnamon.
4. Continue to cook for an additional 5 minutes, stirring occasionally.
5. Serve hot and topped with chopped almonds for added crunch and iron.

Yogurt Chia Seed Parfait

Ingredients:

- 1/2 cup Greek yogurt
- 1 teaspoon chia seeds
- 1/4 cup fresh berries
- 1 teaspoon honey (optional)

Instructions:

1. In a small bowl, mix together the Greek yogurt and chia seeds.
2. Let it sit for 10-15 minutes to allow the chia seeds to absorb some of the liquid from the yogurt and thicken.
3. Layer the yogurt mixture with fresh berries in a glass or jar.
4. Drizzle honey on top for added sweetness, if desired.
5. Refrigerate for at least 30 minutes before serving to allow flavors to blend together.
6. This parfait can be made ahead of time and stored in the fridge for up to 3 days.

Nourishing Lunches

Chickpea & Cucumber Salad

Ingredients:

- 1 cup canned chickpeas, rinsed
- 1 cucumber, diced
- 1/4 cup fresh parsley, chopped
- Juice of 1 lemon
- 2 tablespoons olive oil
- Salt and pepper to taste

Instructions:

1. Combine chickpeas, cucumber, and parsley in a bowl.
2. Whisk together lemon juice, olive oil, salt, and pepper. Toss with the salad.

Lentil & Sweet Potato Soup

Ingredients:

- 1 cup red lentils
- 1 sweet potato, diced
- 1 onion, chopped
- 2 cups low-sodium vegetable broth
- 1 teaspoon cumin
- 1 tablespoon olive oil

Instructions:

1. Sauté onions in olive oil until soft. Add diced sweet potato and cook for 2 minutes.
2. Stir in lentils, cumin, and vegetable broth. Simmer for 25–30 minutes until lentils and sweet potatoes are tender.

Roasted Veggie & Quinoa Bowl

Ingredients:

- 1/2 cup cooked quinoa
- 1 cup roasted vegetables (zucchini, bell peppers, carrots)
- 2 tablespoons tahini dressing

Instructions:

1. Arrange quinoa and roasted vegetables in a bowl.
2. Drizzle with tahini dressing and toss lightly before eating.

Tofu Stir-Fry with Brown Rice

Ingredients:

- 1/2 block firm tofu, cubed
- 1 cup mixed vegetables (green beans, carrots, onions)
- 1 tablespoon soy sauce
- 1 tablespoon sesame oil
- 1/2 cup cooked brown rice

Instructions:

1. Heat sesame oil in a pan and cook tofu cubes until lightly browned.
2. Add mixed vegetables and cook for 7–8 minutes. Stir in soy sauce and serve over brown rice.

Light, Iron-Smart Dinners

Baked Cod with Zucchini Noodles

Ingredients:

- 1 cod fillet
- 1 zucchini, spiralized
- 1 tablespoon olive oil
- 1/2 teaspoon garlic powder
- Salt and pepper to taste

Instructions:

1. Preheat oven to 375°F (190°C). Rub cod with olive oil, garlic powder, salt, and pepper. Bake for 12–15 minutes.
2. Sauté zucchini noodles in a pan for 2–3 minutes and serve with cod.

Black Bean & Veggie Tacos

Ingredients:

- 1/2 cup black beans, rinsed
- 1 cup mixed vegetables (diced peppers, corn, onions)
- 2 small corn tortillas
- 1 tablespoon salsa

Instructions:

1. Heat black beans and sautéed vegetables in a pan.
2. Spoon the mixture into tortillas and top with salsa.

Grilled Tilapia with Sweet Potato Mash

Ingredients:

- 1 tilapia fillet
- 1 medium sweet potato, boiled and mashed
- 1 teaspoon olive oil
- Salt and pepper to taste

Instructions:

1. Grill tilapia until cooked through (about 3–4 minutes per side).
2. Serve with mashed sweet potato seasoned with olive oil, salt, and pepper.

Lentil & Veggie Pasta

Ingredients:

- 1/2 cup cooked lentils
- 1 cup cooked pasta (non-fortified)
- 1/2 cup sautéed broccoli
- 1 tablespoon olive oil
- 1/2 teaspoon garlic powder

Instructions:

1. Toss cooked pasta with lentils, broccoli, olive oil, and garlic powder.
2. Serve warm as a light, nutritious dinner.

Snacks & Sides

Cucumber & Guacamole Bites

Ingredients:

- 1 cucumber, sliced
- 1/4 cup guacamole

Instructions:

1. Top each cucumber slice with a small spoonful of guacamole.
2. Serve as a healthy and refreshing snack or side dish.

Yogurt & Berry Dip

Ingredients:

- 1/2 cup Greek yogurt
- 1/2 cup mixed fresh berries

Instructions:

1. In a small bowl, mash the fresh berries with a fork.
2. Mix in the Greek yogurt until well combined.
3. Serve as a protein-packed dip for fruit or veggies.

Roasted Chickpeas

Ingredients:

- 1 cup canned chickpeas, rinsed
- 1 tablespoon olive oil
- 1/2 teaspoon paprika

Instructions:

1. Preheat your oven to 400 degrees Fahrenheit.
2. Combine the chickpeas, olive oil, and paprika in a bowl, stirring until they are evenly coated.
3. Spread the chickpeas on a baking sheet lined with parchment paper.
4. Bake for 20-25 minutes or until crispy.
5. Let cool before serving as a crunchy and protein-rich snack.

Hummus with Veggie Sticks

Ingredients:

- 1/2 cup hummus
- Sliced celery, bell peppers, or carrots

Instructions:

1. Fill a small bowl with hummus.
2. Wash and slice your choice of vegetables into sticks.
3. Dip the vegetable sticks into the hummus for a healthy and satisfying snack.
4. Optional: Sprinkle some paprika or other spices on top of the hummus for added flavor.

Refreshing Drinks & Teas

Iced Green Tea with Mint

Ingredients:

- 2 green tea bags
- 4 cups boiled water
- Fresh mint leaves
- Ice cubes

Instructions:

1. Steep tea bags and mint leaves in boiled water for 5 minutes.
2. Cool, pour over ice, and serve.

Lemon Ginger Water

Ingredients:

- 4 cups water
- 1 lemon, sliced
- 1-inch piece of ginger

Instructions:

1. Combine water, lemon slices, and ginger in a pitcher.
2. Refrigerate for at least 4 hours or overnight.
3. Serve over ice.

Berry Herbal Tea

Ingredients:

- 2 cups boiling water
- 2 berry-infused herbal tea bags

Instructions:

1. Steep tea bags in boiling water for 5 minutes.
2. Remove tea bags and pour tea into the ice cube tray.
3. Freeze until solid.
4. Use berry herbal tea ice cubes to add flavor to regular water or other beverages.

Cucumber & Lime Sparkling Water

Ingredients:

- 1 liter sparkling water
- 1/2 cucumber, sliced
- 1 lime, sliced

Instructions:

1. In a pitcher, combine sparkling water, sliced cucumber, and sliced lime.
2. Chill in the refrigerator for at least 1 hour.
3. Serve over ice.

These recipes are easy, flavorful, and tailored to support your well-being. Mix and match them to fit your schedule, enhance your energy, and make eating low-iron meals hassle-free!

Lifestyle Tips for Better Management

Living with hemochromatosis calls for a balanced approach to your overall lifestyle, not just diet alone. This chapter offers practical advice to help you improve your well-being and manage symptoms more effectively. By focusing on physical activity, stress management, sleep quality, and knowing when to seek medical advice, you can create a healthier and more manageable routine.

Physical Activity and Fatigue

Physical activity plays a vital role in supporting overall health, especially when managing hemochromatosis. The right exercise routine can boost energy levels, improve circulation, reduce stiffness, and enhance emotional well-being.

However, with the added challenge of fatigue often associated with iron overload, it's crucial to strike a balance between staying active and avoiding overexertion. This section provides practical tips, examples of restorative movement, and encouragement to help you stay active while respecting your energy levels.

Practical Tips for Staying Active

1. **Start Small and Go Gentle:**

   If fatigue is a frequent issue, ease into movement to avoid overwhelming your body. Gentle activities, like a 10–15 minute walk around your neighborhood or simple stretching at home, can have a significant impact. Walking after meals not only helps with digestion but also provides a noticeable energy boost. Even light movement can leave you feeling more refreshed than staying sedentary.

2. **Focus on Low-Impact Exercises:**

   Activities like yoga, swimming, and cycling are ideal as they strengthen muscles and improve circulation without stressing your body. Swimming, in particular, can be fantastic for relieving stiff joints and cooling your body, offering a soothing full-body workout. Yoga and cycling, whether outdoors or on a stationary bike, allow you to control intensity based on how you're feeling that day.

3. **Explore Strength Training Safely:**

   Building muscle can support better energy management and promote overall physical endurance.

If you're new to strength training, start small. Bodyweight exercises like squats, modified planks, or push-ups are low-risk and help build foundational strength. Resistance bands are also effective for guided and gentle strength-building. Over time, you can progress to light hand weights, focusing on proper form and controlled movements to prevent strain.

4. **Pay Attention to Your Body:**

Your body knows best, so don't ignore its signals. If you feel unusually drained or fatigued, give yourself permission to rest. Pushing through tiredness can lead to worsened fatigue, leaving you less able to stay consistent with your physical activity routine. It's okay to take things slow and pick up where you left off when your energy returns.

Restorative Movement Ideas

1. **Gentle Yoga Poses:**

Certain yoga poses work wonders for stretching tight muscles and calming both mind and body. Poses like child's pose, downward dog, cat-cow stretches, or lying twists relieve tension in your back and shoulders while encouraging relaxation. Look for beginner yoga classes or free online videos that guide you through gentle flows suitable for all levels.

2. **Tai Chi for Meditation and Motion:**

   Tai chi is a meditative practice combining deliberate, slow movements with focused breathing. This ancient form of exercise improves circulation, balance, and flexibility while calming the mind. Even ten minutes a day can help you feel more relaxed and grounded.

3. **Stretching or Light Mobility Exercises:**

   Incorporating stretches into your daily routine helps maintain flexibility and circulation, especially if you spend long periods seated. Stretch your arms, neck, legs, and lower back gently throughout the day to prevent stiffness from setting in. Light exercises like shoulder rolls or gentle arm circles are great for regaining energy.

4. **Walking for Functional Fitness:**

   A simple walk is one of the most accessible forms of activity and can be adjusted based on how you're feeling. A walk around the block at a leisurely pace is perfect for easing fatigue, while a brisker stroll can elevate your heart rate if you're feeling more energized.

Consistency Over Intensity

Consistency, not intensity, is the key to reaping the benefits of physical activity when managing hemochromatosis. Instead of pushing yourself to the limit or hitting the gym every day, prioritize small, regular bouts of movement that align with your energy levels.

- *Set Realistic Goals*: Aim to move for 10–20 minutes per day, whether that's walking, yoga, or gentle stretching. Even short sessions done consistently add up to real progress over time.
- *Create a Routine*: Establish a routine that fits naturally into your lifestyle, such as doing light yoga every morning or taking an evening walk after dinner. This helps movement feel less like a chore and more like a seamless part of your day.
- *Track How You Feel*: Journal your energy levels before and after movement to identify which types of activities help you feel more energized versus drained. This can help you tailor your routine to your unique needs.

It's easy to get discouraged if fatigue feels like it's holding you back, but remember that every small effort toward moving your body counts. Consistent gentle activity not only supports your physical health but can also reduce mental sluggishness, lift your mood, and improve your sleep quality. Over time, you'll likely notice a positive shift in how you feel daily.

Celebrate small wins in your wellness journey, like a walk or yoga session, as they reflect your commitment to health. Pair exercise with balanced nutrition, proper sleep, and rest days for a holistic approach to managing hemochromatosis and boosting energy and quality of life.

Stress, Sleep, and Iron Regulation

Living with hemochromatosis involves more than just monitoring your diet and exercise routine. Chronic stress and poor sleep can interfere with your body's ability to regulate iron levels, potentially worsening symptoms like fatigue, irritability, and overall discomfort.

Finding ways to manage stress and improve sleep hygiene is key to maintaining balance and enhancing your quality of life. This section provides actionable tips and insights into how stress, sleep, and iron regulation are intertwined.

Managing Stress

Stress is a normal part of life, but chronic, unmanaged stress can trigger inflammation in your body. For individuals managing hemochromatosis, inflammation can influence how iron is absorbed and stored, potentially exacerbating symptoms. By prioritizing stress management, you can help your body function more effectively while improving your mental and emotional well-being.

1. **Practice Mindfulness:**

    Mindfulness techniques, such as meditation, deep breathing, or progressive muscle relaxation, are excellent tools for calming the mind and body. Mindfulness meditation encourages you to focus on the present moment, grounding yourself and reducing anxiety.

- ***Example Exercise***: Try the 4-7-8 breathing technique. Breathe in for 4 seconds, hold your breath for 7 seconds, and exhale for 8 seconds. Repeat this cycle 4–5 times. This simple practice can be done anywhere, whether you're at home or taking a quick break during a busy day.

2. **Set Boundaries and Realistic Expectations:**

Constantly juggling too many responsibilities can lead to mental and physical strain. Learn to say no to tasks or commitments that stretch you too thin. Delegating work or asking for help with daily responsibilities can free up time and energy for self-care and relaxation. Remember, protecting your well-being is not selfish; it's essential for long-term health.

3. **Take Short Restorative Breaks:**

Small, intentional breaks during the day can lower stress levels and help prevent burnout. Use your breaks to do something enjoyable, like stepping outside to breathe in fresh air, listening to soothing music, or jotting down your thoughts in a journal. These moments of pause can clear your mind and re-energize you.

4. **Engage in Activities You Enjoy:**

   Dedicate time to hobbies or activities that bring you happiness. Whether it's gardening, painting, yoga, or simply reading, doing something you love offers natural stress relief and allows you to recharge.

Improving Sleep Quality

Sleep is fundamental to healing and restoration, but poor sleep habits can worsen fatigue and disrupt the hormones that regulate your body's iron absorption. Prioritizing good sleep hygiene can make a significant difference in how you feel day to day.

1. **Establish a Sleep Schedule:**

   Create a consistent routine by going to bed and waking up at the same time every day, even on weekends. A regular sleep schedule not only supports hormonal balance but also trains your body to recognize when it's time to rest. This helps prevent long nights of tossing and turning.

2. **Create a Relaxing Environment:**

   Your bedroom should be a calming space conducive to sleep. Keep the room cool, dark, and free of distractions like clutter and electronic devices.

   - *Pro Tips*: Use blackout curtains to reduce external light and a white noise machine to mask disruptive sounds. If your mind tends to race at bedtime, consider keeping a notebook nearby to jot down thoughts and clear your head.

3. **Limit Screen Time Before Bed:**

   Blue light from electronic devices suppresses melatonin production, the hormone needed for sleep. To optimize rest, avoid screens such as phones, tablets, or laptops at least an hour before bedtime. Instead, use that time for quiet, screen-free activities like reading, listening to soft music, or meditating.

4. **Wind Down with Herbal Teas:**

   Certain herbal teas can promote relaxation and improve your nighttime routine. Chamomile, valerian root, and lavender tea are excellent choices for their calming properties. Sip them while engaging in a restful activity, like journaling or light stretching, to prepare your mind and body for sleep.

How Stress and Sleep Affect Iron Regulation

Chronic stress and inadequate sleep can interfere with the body's ability to regulate iron levels. Here's a deeper dive into the connection:

1. **The Impact of Stress:**

    Chronic stress elevates cortisol levels, which can lead to inflammation in the body. This inflammation may affect how iron is absorbed and stored, contributing to imbalances that exacerbate symptoms of hemochromatosis. High stress can also worsen feelings of fatigue and irritability, compounding the challenges of managing iron overload.

2. **The Role of Sleep:**

    Poor sleep limits your body's ability to repair and restore itself overnight. Sleep deprivation also keeps cortisol levels elevated, further affecting inflammation and metabolic processes, including iron regulation. Additionally, lack of sleep directly contributes to physical and mental exhaustion, making it harder to stick to important health routines like healthy eating and exercise.

3. **The Ripple Effect of Balance:**

    Addressing stress and sleep creates positive outcomes across your health. With lower cortisol and inflammation levels, your body has a better chance of regulating iron absorption and minimizing its harmful buildup. Improved sleep also boosts energy levels, helping you manage fatigue and stay consistent with lifestyle changes.

Taking care of your mental health and sleep habits doesn't have to involve big, overwhelming changes. Small, intentional tweaks can make a world of difference. For example, committing to five minutes of mindfulness or drinking herbal tea before bed can help foster better routines over time.

Remember that mental and physical health are deeply connected. By addressing stress and prioritizing restful, high-quality sleep, you're supporting your body's natural ability to function at its best. These steps might seem simple, but their impact on your iron regulation and overall well-being is profound. Be patient with yourself as you build new habits and celebrate every positive change along the way.

When to Talk to Your Doctor

Regular check-ins with your healthcare provider are a critical part of managing hemochromatosis. Be proactive about staying informed and addressing any concerns to prevent complications.

1. **Symptoms That Warrant Immediate Attention:**
   - Extreme fatigue or weakness that doesn't improve with rest.
   - Joint pain, especially if it worsens over time.
   - Persistent abdominal pain could indicate liver complications.
   - A sudden change in symptoms, such as dizziness, rapid heartbeat, or unexplained weight loss.
2. **Routine Monitoring:**
   - Follow your doctor's recommendations for regular blood tests to monitor ferritin levels and ensure treatment is effective.
   - Share any changes in your diet, activity levels, or symptoms during visits to provide a complete health picture.
3. **Discuss Treatment Options:**
   - If you're struggling to manage iron levels through diet and treatment (such as phlebotomy), discuss alternative approaches or additional interventions with your doctor.
   - A personalized plan may include medication, specialized dietary adjustments, or referral to a nutritionist.
4. **Address Emotional Well-Being:**

   Living with a chronic condition can impact mental health. If you're feeling overwhelmed, anxious, or depressed, reach out to your doctor. They can connect you with counseling or support resources suited to your needs.

5. **Preventive Care:**

   Your healthcare provider can help screen for and prevent complications related to hemochromatosis, such as diabetes, liver disease, or heart issues, through regular appointments and early interventions.

By integrating small, thoughtful changes into your lifestyle and staying consistent with medical care, you can better manage hemochromatosis while prioritizing your health and well-being. Keep track of your progress, celebrate your successes, and remain open to adjusting your routines as needed for long-term success.

Conclusion

Thank you for taking the time to explore this guide on managing hemochromatosis. By completing it, you've already taken an important step toward understanding how to manage this condition and protect your long-term health. Learning to live with hemochromatosis may feel challenging at first, but remember, you are not alone, and a healthier, balanced lifestyle is within your reach.

One key takeaway from this guide is the power of knowledge and planning. Understanding the role of diet in controlling iron levels is crucial. By implementing strategies such as limiting iron-rich foods, choosing inhibitors like calcium, and timing your meals wisely, you can make significant strides in managing your condition. The sample meal plans, grocery lists, and cooking tips provided are there to empower you with practical solutions. With these tools, you can still enjoy a satisfying and flavorful diet without feeling restricted.

Lifestyle adjustments are equally vital. Beyond food, finding balance in areas like physical activity, stress management, and sleep will enhance your overall well-being. Hemochromatosis can affect your energy levels and mood, but by listening to your body and making small, sustainable changes, you can reduce fatigue, improve your day-to-day life, and find strength in routine.

It's also important to advocate for your own health. Regular check-ins with your doctor and communicating any changes in your symptoms will help prevent complications. Your healthcare providers are there to guide you, but as someone living with this condition, you are the most important member of your care team. Ask questions. Speak up about challenges. You know your body better than anyone else.

Remember, managing hemochromatosis isn't about perfection; it's about progress. Some days will feel easier than others, and that's okay. Celebrate your wins, no matter how small they may seem. Whether it's successfully sticking to meal prep or finding an afternoon to take a relaxing walk, these moments matter. Each step you take brings you closer to a lifestyle that works for both you and your health.

If there's one piece of advice to take away, it's this: focus on what's within your control. You can decide what to put on your plate, how to spend your time, and when to rest or reach out for support. These decisions may feel like small actions, but over time, they add up to big changes. By staying proactive and making informed choices, you are setting yourself up for a healthier, happier future.

Finally, be kind to yourself. Managing a chronic condition isn't easy, but with persistence and the right mindset, you can create a life that feels balanced and fulfilling. You've taken the time to educate yourself, and that effort alone is something to be proud of.

Frequently Asked Questions (FAQs)

Should I Take Supplements?

If you have hemochromatosis, be very careful with supplements. Avoid all iron supplements or multivitamins that include iron, as they can worsen iron overload. Additionally, steer clear of high doses of vitamin C supplements, as they increase how much iron your body absorbs. Always read the labels carefully and consult your doctor before taking any kind of supplement, even common ones. A healthcare provider can determine if you need a specific vitamin or mineral, like magnesium or vitamin D, based on your overall health.

What Blood Tests Should I Monitor?

Several important blood tests can help track your iron levels:

- ***Ferritin Test***: This measures the amount of stored iron in your body. High levels typically indicate excess iron.

- *Transferrin Saturation*: This test shows how much iron is attached to transferrin, a protein that moves iron through your blood. Elevated percentages suggest iron overload.
- *Liver Tests*: These can check for any liver problems caused by too much iron.
- *Hemoglobin and Hematocrit*: These tests look for anemia or irregularities in red blood cell levels, which can develop during treatment.

Keep up with regular blood tests as recommended by your doctor to make sure your treatment is working well and your iron levels are in check.

Can This Diet Help My Other Symptoms?

Yes, following a low-iron diet can help more than just your iron levels. By lowering iron-rich foods and focusing on fresh vegetables, whole grains, and plant-based proteins, you can ease symptoms like fatigue, joint pain, and stomach discomfort. These healthier food choices can also help protect your heart and liver from future complications. Many people report improved energy, less inflammation, and better digestion when sticking to a balanced, low-iron eating plan.

What About Vegetarian or Vegan Diets?

A vegetarian or vegan diet can work well when managing hemochromatosis because it avoids heme iron, which is found in meats and is absorbed more easily by the body. Non-heme iron found in plant foods is harder for the body to absorb, which is beneficial. Still, you need to watch out for overloading on plant-based sources of iron, like spinach, lentils, and fortified cereals. Pair these foods with calcium-rich options or tannin-containing beverages (like tea or coffee) to lower iron absorption. Consulting with a nutritionist can help you stay balanced and healthy on a plant-based diet.

Can I Drink Alcohol?

Alcohol should be limited when you have hemochromatosis, especially if you have any liver-related complications. Alcohol can intensify the damage caused by excess iron in the liver. If you choose to drink, do so in moderation and follow any specific guidelines from your doctor. Reducing alcohol intake can help protect your liver and overall health.

How Often Should I Donate Blood?

Blood donation is often a key treatment for managing iron levels, called therapeutic phlebotomy. How often you need to donate depends on your ferritin levels and your doctor's recommendations. Some people may need to donate weekly at first, while others might only require it every few months once their levels stabilize. Always follow the schedule set by your doctor, as too few or too many donations could harm your health.

Are There Any Foods I Should Completely Avoid?

Certain foods like organ meats, iron-fortified products, and undercooked shellfish are high in iron and can pose risks for individuals with hemochromatosis. Limiting other high-iron foods like red meats and pairing iron-rich meals with inhibitors such as dairy or tea can also help manage your iron intake effectively.

References and Helpful Links

Nichols, H. (2024, January 24). Everything you need to know about the hemochromatosis diet.
https://www.medicalnewstoday.com/articles/hemochromatosis-diet

Ms, E. L. (2023, February 22). The best diet for hemochromatosis. Healthline. https://www.healthline.com/health/hemochromatosis-diet

Hereditary hemochromatosis: MedlinePlus Genetics. (n.d.). https://medlineplus.gov/genetics/condition/hereditary-hemochromatosis/#:~:text=Type%201%20hemochromatosis%20results%20from,gene%20cause%20type%204%20hemochromatosis.

Rd, V. T., PhD. (2023, April 24). How to Increase the Absorption of Iron from Foods. Healthline.
https://www.healthline.com/nutrition/increase-iron-absorption

Iron, transferrin, ferritin and total iron-binding capacity - Uniprix. (n.d.). Uniprix.
https://www.uniprix.com/en/article/laboratory-tests/iron-transferrin-ferritin-and-total-iron-binding-capacity#:~:text=Transferrin%20is%20correlated%20with%20total,marrow%2C%20spleen%2C%20and%20muscles.

Christiansen, S. (2025, April 9). Hemochromatosis diet. Verywell Health. https://www.verywellhealth.com/hemochromatosis-diet-4774139

Hemochromatosis Help. (2020, October 23). Hemochromatosis recipes | Hemochromatosis help. https://hemochromatosishelp.com/recipes/

www.ingramcontent.com/pod-product-compliance
Lightning Source LLC
LaVergne TN
LVHW012030060526
838201LV00061B/4535